ANTHOLOGY ATRIUMS
BOOK TWO

Copyright © 2025 by Anthony P. Prior

All rights reserved.

No part of this book may be reproduced or used in any manner without written permission of the copyright owner except for the use of quotations in a book review.
For more information,
contact: tpriorart@aol.com

FIRST EDITION

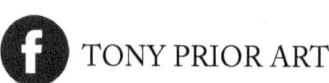 TONY PRIOR ART

ISBN: 978-1-80541-730-9 (paperback)
ISBN: 978-1-80541-729-3 (ebook)

ANTHOLOGY ATRIUMS

BOOK TWO

ANTHONY P PRIOR

TABLE OF CONTENTS

Hash-tag#	1
Keep Setup	2
Time Again	3
Not Caput	4
Forefathers	5
Same Thing	6
Good Is Bad	7
Next Wave	8
Getting it Right	9
Pending	10
Projecting How I Feel	11
Ulterior Motives	12
Block	13
Needing Space	14
Get Criticism	15

Do Without	16
Persisted	17
Make it Happen	18
Choice Of Words	19
Think For Myself	20
Taken Seriously	22
I'll Get Back To You	23
Resilient	24
Temperamental	25
This Dystopian Hell	26
No Going Back	27
Glitch	28
Bus Load Of Faith	29
Good Stuff	30
Coiled Spring	31
Got My Heart	32
Time Is Slipping	33

Up With New	34
Get It Right	35
Whole Gamut	36
Raw Edge	37
Saving Grace	38
Art Space	39
All In The Planning	40
Consideration	41
Others' Point Of View	42
Occupied Mind	43
Keep In Touch with The Digital World	44
Too Much	45
Revisited	46
Elemental	47
Abstraction	48

HASH-TAG#

Line repeating#,
Chorus line singing#,
Over again and again#,
Subtitles repeating#,
Line of a song ding dong#,
Over and over#,
Same again#,
Repetition#,
Prompting next move#,
Chess piece#,
Pawn-king4#,
Castle-knight-castling#,
Next round? #
Same again#,
Suits you sir#,
Carry if off#,
#drawings Instagram,
@online#,
Making a hash of it#,
Complicit carryon#,
All together now#,
Pulling it off#,
Once more for the boys#,
What again#.

KEEP SETUP

Don't change a thing,
It has worked so far so keep it,
Change rearranges my mind unkind,
Adapted to things all along same old song,
New isn't always better to the letter,
Tried upgrading got things all wrong,
Thinking I was with it, better without,
Thought I had to spend to mend,
I had already got it simple rearrange,
Repositioning repurposed my condition,
This seemed new contributing to,
Change is as good as a rest contest,
Saved myself lots of money being straight,
Looking back couldn't contemplate or,
Navigate my way around different sound,
Am I a bit autistic with my playlist?
Think I could be simplistic unfortunate,
I like to know where I am plain same,
Occasionally change picture frame keep sane.

TIME AGAIN

I would learn different languages,
Words come back to haunt me,
Bits of French, allez dans le rue de Gard,
I live on Station Road, uncannily ironically,
I would also wish I'd paid attention to,
My Latin class, which now seems to be,
The basis for our English language.
In Bara tum Dae belly fruit,
Roman numerals X1x11,
All seems to be making senescence now,
Didn't during school, non comprenez,
I was narrow minded all seemed foreign,
There seemed too much to take in,
Information overload silly old toad,
Teacher preacher didn't reach me,
I would now love to be able to speak,
A foreign language fluently go abroad,
Show off how eloquent intelligent I am,
Speaking at restaurants "Tres bon monsieur,"
Combien - d'ici ? pour le extravaganza,
I would be fluent generous perfect comrade,
They would think how nice the English are,
A perfect example of our friendship,
Entente cordial.

NOT CAPUT

Had it, had my day, knackered,
Finished, old, not in touch, distant,
Life in the old dog, has been, done for,
Got hope, optimistic, light end of tunnel,
Never say die, senile old fart, waster,
Grown old, rest on laurels, time to quit,
Silver surfer, pensioned off, retired,
Done it all, experienced, learnt from mistakes,
Old timer, no quitter, well-travelled,
Tell youth a thing or two, reserved,
Seen it all before, memories cherished,
History repeats, remember well,
Still got my faculties, presence of mind,
Save the day, not giving away
Respect duty, law of the land,
Moral duty act upon, donate,
Helping hand, with it, sharp as,
Spirit is willing, always wanted,
Expect too much, one day,
Planned to, fallen by, shy,
Correct me please, got it wrong,
Second chance, new romance,
Let diligent diligence commence.

FOREFATHERS

I have memories of grandparents,
Norman and Nel at Priors Garage,
They ran Grandads car repair business,
Norman was adventurous forward thinking,
Granny ran the family children my dad,
His brothers, sister, and local methodist,
Church, Uncle Tom Cobly and all,
Their garage was a hive for passing folk,
There was petrol pump filling station,
No money in it granddad would say,
Local Land and gentry would go elsewhere if,
He put his prices up, uncles wearing flat caps,
Worked in the garage, a sense of comradery,
Was present all for one, grandad would say.
Go and tell your granny the wars over and,
Could he have another biscuit with his cuppa,
They talked about Hat common local Lord,
Going on holiday to Dorset Bridport Gundry's,
Gave us kids a stick of rock to suck,
He marvelled about fossils collected,
From the rock face a collection of,
Ammonites, history telling all way back,
A sense of owning and possessing the past.

SAME THING

Done it again setup transcribes,
What's wrong is correct but contrite,
The difference hasn't been adjusted,
Malpractice bound to happen once more,
Having to correct defect by default,
Same thing will happen again set out,
Is originally right but not adapted,
To continue needs correcting format,
The formula plan is too rigid structure,
I want flexible ease to create please,
Both ways say change pattern plan,
Equate equation inclusive brackets,
Balance relaxed with advanced,
Backwards forwards commence stop,
Deliberate derivative forceful fortunate,
Inconclusive conclusions introduced,
Abashed embarrassments ashamed,
Financial deficits afraid paid,
Contribution give and take,
Profit and loss accounts accounted.

GOOD IS BAD

Definitely sad not glad reverse roles,
Anarchy lovely hate grate mate darling,
Pushed too far near and distant,
Opposites attract bearing no fact,
Plus, minus contrary defines,
Reminds blind clear as a bell,
Heaven goes to hell as far as I can tell,
Be quiet yell shut your face no grace,
Quickly now set the pace slowly,
Vacant vague positive negative,
Harassed at ease F off friend,
Absent without leave relieve retrieve,
Fiction fact detract giveaway,
Subliminal obvious contrary full-on,
Aesthetic subjective opinion unclear,
Beautiful ugly personal taste,
Objective too subjective lost directive,
Fragrance unfamiliar stinks,
Fresh manure lovely smell,
Bittersweet shit not a bit of it,
Dancing prancing twill twirl,
Begger's belief percolated,
Infirm flexible good turn.

NEXT WAVE

Of course, waiting I'll get up on the next one,
Several have passed me by not right,
A good one is full of potential rising,
Sunk down in a trough momentum surges,
Picked up after backing up on surf topper,
Powerful arm grabs hold green looking down,
Experience says this will do steady true,
Collecting gather rising acting play stay,
Steady eddy in control good stance,
Loving what I'm doing solid romance,
Pushed up erect know good effect,
Balanced moves shifting weight gate,
State of lift away surge converge,
Correct shuffle power humbled,
Speed relative to collective,
Still alive contrive fresh air fare,
A thrill then spills dunked salty drill,
Act one solution solved hard landing,
In deep neap tide along for ride complied.

GETTING IT RIGHT

Of course, we all do our best,
Follow rules of the road,
Start our daily routine normally,
Change, stand corrected adapted,
As input sets different course,
Selected chosen interesting,
Pick of what's on offer challenging,
Surveyed not sure about anything,
Choice is mine difficult define combine,
Must revert back to what used to do,
Often sure can do don't want to,
Got to believe committed retrieve,
Do it again can't refrain same,
Blame it on bored ignored,
Must freshen up invent new,
Turn things around sound,
Project project profusely,
Be generous easy on yourself,
Let cars pullout before you,
Defy bullish command,
Harmonious harmony harmless,
Prodigious penalties pointless,
Give and take rewards,
Efficient ergonomic way.

PENDING

Its always pending waiting for it to happen,
Returns, payment, acknowledgement, decision,
Ok, most things are getting quicker with Ai,
Anticipating my next move, needing approving,
My solution being impatient is keep busy.
I must be good at multitasking changing,
Difficult to keep track of outstanding,
Order of jobs in line to do crossed off,
Belligerent persistent queue jumpers,
Faster-faster, waiting belating put off,
Tasks hindered delegated reminded,
Shuffle the pack answering back,
No joke bespoke random answers,
Suggest contest against apprehend,
Pat-pending don't copy around bend,
Regulations defer efficiency imminent,
No right to produce rearrange,
Change design set pattern pending,
Safeguard patent issued protected.

PROJECTING HOW I FEEL

Can people really see how I feel?
I look at other people's faces to judge,
You can usually see what mood,
Happy sad glad alright not bad,
It's always important to perceive,
Before entering conversation,
Once acknowledged I'm away,
Broken down all barriers now proceed,
Questioned health wealth careful stealth,
The art of conversation skilful hopeful,
Converse is worth by return response,
Entered engaged displayed said,
Start repouring soon all for candour,
Productive proactive produces platitude,
Punctually duality forming a bond in kind,
Reasonable reasoning rational collaborate,
Converse shows its worth priceless,
Harmonious harmony decisive,
Deliberate discussion proves poignant,
Positive production hits home,
Being understood all for the good,
Being on a level is all convivial,
Trust in others to deliver revival.

ULTERIOR MOTIVES

Lying beneath alternative point beyond,
Different outcome envisaged seen hoped,
There seems to be a political motion leading,
A personal subjective reasoning reason,
Deceiving deception sort conceived made,
Portrayed outcome misconceived believed,
Subliminal directive directing the equation,
End goal already made getting there devious,
Masquerades covered up taken a set course,
To deliver promiscuous pretentious promises,
Devious deviation delivering said deception,
Conception conceived considerable application,
Applied to momentous augmented argument,
Seeing both sides wanting to deliver poignant,
Opinion as to how this should turn out,
Laid out planned out afore said made up for,
Wrongs already committed that can't,
Be undone guilty as charged m'lord.

BLOCK

Sometimes my mind goes blank,
Can't think what to do have got stuck,
It might be writers block no way to turn,
I'm looking for something waiting,
I suppose I've got to make it happen,
Its up to me to get inventive organise,
Move problems out of the way unblock,
First must realise what the problem is,
Seeing the restriction malfunction,
Get my mojo working.
What has relieved is respected,
Other people's good work subjected,
See how I can help with reciprocation,
I must now follow in return with a,
Good commendation reviews true blue,
Only fair to respond with good compare,
They have eased the way I must with,
All decency respond correctly well done!
Now feel like a block party invite everybody.

NEEDING SPACE

We have booked a holiday away,
Just thinking about it expands my view,
Watched a video layout of pools views,
Had the right effect uplifted the depressed,
Sullen sunken abandoned ship now afloat,
The capsized derided unfounded found,
Ready to play the part try on new can do,
Exotic erotic suncream glean screen scene,
Evolving away from stay-at-home stop,
Pack up put up getting in the groove,
My record had got stuck repetitive tune,
Thoughtful resolution imbued rings true,
Get ready a lot to do finish resolve,
Got to get my head around new profound,
Consider considerate left behind,
Have made allowances forgive allowed,
Each to their own safe and sound,
Space has been found share new ground.

GET CRITICISM

Yes, I get it does affect me absolutely,
Whether being misunderstood or for the good,
Or bad ignorance has its place in the race,
No disgrace its common place actual,
I must listen digest accept draw on,
All part of life's conundrum,
I can feel hurt from simple remarks,
So have to quickly defend,
Make amends quip back quickly,
Smart retort levels field,
From which I can yield,
Obstinate view how seen,
Don't want must change,
Listened to extremes,
Pitch somewhere in between,
Cajaole their prison sentence,
Augment accept relent argument,
Repent only if true,
Can be seen as tic-Ardy-boo,
Point taken pitch elsewhere only fair,
Considerable consideration considered,
If only they would tolerate my word,
Not always right little contrite,
I've heard defend my way,
Try to change rearrange,
Accept theirs isn't absolutely,
Mine is defiant politely!

DO WITHOUT

Ok, getting personal now, I can't,
Why should I life is for living so live it,
Worked hard for bread and butter not a nutter!
It takes a lot of self-discipline to stop smoking,
Kind of drug taste hit get off on it need feed,
The solution to addiction is to see alternative,
Needs can offer better response without,
False pretentions wrong directions,
Giving up a collective decision from,
Within reasoning pro's cons to gain,
Momentum will-power to stand against,
Self-inflicted destructive limp harassment,
Don't be such a wimp relying on a whim,
Chastise yourself improverished wealth,
Just to sustain a neurotic gain see yourself,
As pathetic apathetic ruination of,
Beautiful life health be true to yourself,
Can do better must give-up wonder lust,
Antisocial behaviour gets with it buster,
Stop contrary fairy be decent don't decent.

PERSISTED

I had a problem with computer program,
Got advice from know-all, oh yes of course!
How many times have I got to tell you!
Reprimanded I continue abashed,
I have got to learn wrong generation,
Its simple when you know,
Paying attention now try it out,
Trying to remember what to do,
It seems all wrong but carryon,
Open two versions of the same,
Highlight text copy paste,
Yes, it's worked now save,
Now know where I am,
Sorted the problem myself,
Confidence grows good health.
Sticky wicket good turn learnt,
Wrong then right turned out alright,
Listened to advise muddled through,
Got to keep trying don't give up!

MAKE IT HAPPEN

To start the day with get it straight in my head,
From a list of jobs to chase up,
Obvious importance to must do,
Research possible helpers' availability,
Must phone hospital, impossible,
Left message impractical hopeful,
Have researched on a list must persist,
Self-important must wait your turn yawn,
Impatient patient persists ahead of lists,
Trying to find a way through have to,
Speak to administrator making a check,
Message left now defect differences,
Now change tack change of line,
Think of other interests to pursue,
Other interest's jobs needing assistance,
I can think of other things to do,
But singularly only my main goal rings true,
Obsessive compulsive direct main effect,
Have pushed the limits now back on transit.

CHOICE OF WORDS

I must choose carefully for fear of saying the
Wrong thing being misundestood,
It's easy to get it wrong come across as blunt,
Tactless cause crude rude misconstrued,
Taken the wrong way alternative delivery,
Pronunciation can literally confuse issues,
Sounds wrong got it wrong not clear,
Also, double meanings same but different,
Spring water, spring tide, spring to your feet,
Sprinkle, sprinkled, sprinkler, spring season,
Springer, coiled spring, spring sprung, springs,
Bed springs, spring in your stride, spring bank
Holiday, spring in your shoes, springtime,
Watch spring, spring greens, spring flowers,
Springtime of the year, springy deflection,
Springboard, spring off the tongue, spring,
Daffodils, step into spring, spring bounce,
Spring it to you, spring off one-another,
Spring it on you, clock spring, car springs.

THINK FOR MYSELF

Big boy now doesn't need help,
Happy with my settings surroundings,
Secure able to work produce,
Keep it simple within reach,
Get myself organised ready,
For anything anytime,
Presentable presence of mind,
Setup level start suitable job,
Depending on correct incentive,
Thinking how to proceed,
Things to do what's needed,
Stop thinking of myself,
Others need help,
Must concede give-up greed,
Adapt to always taking,
Generous partaking,
Defect reflect connect,
Thoughtlessness stubborn,
Automatic doing,
Change resolve,

Can be generous,
Towards most,
Don't think of cost,
Altruistic effective,
Good subjective,
Connect reflective,
Deflect demands,
Singular objective,
Making doing,
All enjoying,
Pleasure reciprocated,
Back on myself,
For giving up wealth,
Of ideas commandeered
Knowledge is free,
Experience tells,
Give-up sales talk,
Go for walk,
Over and beyond,
Friendly correspond,
A helping hand,
Expands friends,
When make amends,
Comprehend.

TAKEN SERIOUSLY

Came as a surprise interest in my work,
Old paintings done at college,
Must be back in fashion expressionism,
Come around not realised back then,
I've kept old work attached can't throw,
How do you price? Don't want to part,
Not going cheap going to keep,
Got to find out how much it's desired,
Or is it just a wind come to find,
Trickery might be playing a part,
Tread carefully avoids dodgy,
Suspicions of too fantastic,
Probably wanting to steal my plastic,
Been bitten before once no more,
Only trust in confidence must,
Believable unbelievable,
Contentious plausible confess,
Too good to be true can't do,
Nearly fell for dramatic fall.

I'LL GET BACK TO YOU

Just getting started is an ordeal too much,
Checking messages apparent pledges,
Confessing, more or Lessing demanding,
Apprehending unknown condescending,
Want to get on with thought consideration,
I've got my own plans desires contrivers,
Fighting through misconstructed follow through,
A lot to do want to can't do probable should,
Being held back by overzealous apparitions,
Got to keep it simple steps in line confine,
Pushing too hard gets baffled blinded,
Then when I've sieved through what to do,
Difficulties disappear construction reappears,
With no fear of repetition dereliction confuse,
Dismissing all to abundant redundant ideas,
Set back in arrears left behind only to remind,
Of unfortunate adventures promiscuous,
Proposals present problems irreversible,
So, I promise to get back to your digeridoo,
That will do, confirm said to do.

RESILIENT

I've had a cold which has knocked the stuffing,
Out of me, lost all stamina joints weak creaking,
Knowing I'll get through this coughing spitting,
Body aching lost rhythem back out only pout,
Tripping walking difficult thinking of nowt,
Clear thoughts count to noughts,
Dizzy pathetic apology nonsensical,
However still thinking doable done,
Have a backlog of jobs to do stuck,
Lost my flow doing well below,
Throat sore suck tablet roll around,
Nearly choke lost swallowed,
Concentrate on deliberate,
All my time spent on survive,
Handicapped staying alive,
Drama say's do or die.
Feeling immortal strive,
Hope keeps me going,
Incredible research,
Helps with my resilience.

TEMPERAMENTAL

A bit iffy unreliable changeable,
Artistic talent with variations,
Makeup ephemeral uncertain,
Far too talented for own good,
Swing in favour of then back,
Dependent correct procedure,
Keep in good books assuredly,
Definite definition lost,
Against all odds competes,
Pretentious pretence,
Vague apparition,
Hasten fortuitously,
Deferred negotiation,
Ambiguous conclusion,
For better or worse,
Assured winner loses,
Happen upon accident,
Winner takes all,
Occasion could be better.

THIS DYSTOPIAN HELL

Side of life to shock When I watch news on Tv
they show the worst, get attention.
"You might find,
Some of these scenes upsetting"!
Attention sought 'can't look away!'
Gruesome disturbing realism,
Taken to the front line!
Everything visible by video,
Soldiers interviewed at the front,
Action packed 'Actively Active'.
It is shocking death bombing,
We all know better,
Stop deadly competitor!
Taking sides derides,
All the same but different,
Simplistic relent,
Stops the argument,
Patronise the bigot,
Causing the upset.

NO GOING BACK

Forward is the only way of delivery,
Improvements of efficiency can be made,
To help improve orderly transition change,
Rearrange contents offer new display,
Comparable differences deferred displayed,
Change of inventory reinvented recalculated,
The not so bad sense of sensibility lifts,
My outlook showing bright horizons,
Not thinking of going too far but far enough,
To say I've been away change hither say,
Accommodating different scenes of obscurity,
To reset my mind friend's opinions not before,
I've studied a map. Not going back transition,
Flack adventures mischievous excitedly,
Explore unusual haven't been here before,
Want to see more of the same new picture frame,
Kind of marching on new appraisal singsong,
Taking new breath of fresh air aux compare,
All tributaries leading me to the sea romantically,
Stirred up a soul of enjoyment new enrolment,
To the good life leaving behind strife.

GLITCH

When something doesn't work with,
Your computer electric device it's got a bug,
In the system cross wires faults,
It's malfunctioning not working correctly,
Problematic problem not used to,
Solution is to switch off back on again,
That should solve it resolved,
Back to its default programmed setting,
If that doesn't fix the problem you're stuffed,
Next try to analyse all discrepancies,
Mind over matter does matter,
Try tapping to against hard object,
Maybe even drop it accidently,
These are all proven technical solutions,
Outwit clever engineer's dodgy importers,
Bad copies copied dysfunctional,
Everything is guaranteed for a year,
Doesn't make the problems disappear,
Glad you kept receipt return delete,
Wait in turn money paid delayed.

BUS LOAD OF FAITH

It sure does to get by daily trial,
New challenges appear every day,
Change of situations amended rearranged,
Nothing static must be flexible with people,
We're all trying our best to fit in,
Missed appointments rearranged complain,
Missed out should have done, hindsight,
Forgot to inform of discrepancy apologise,
Tactics of delay pay improvise provisionally,
Trip over own decisions clumsily unfortunately,
Nothing is definite individual subjective,
Making its own way solitary unforgiven,
Answerable to nobody obliged deride,
Sympathize can't abide ignore deplore,
Pressurise pressure applied guilt denied,
Must keep on don't give up rolling along,
Trust in your own intuition to decide.

GOOD STUFF

A matter of quality original,
Second to none, pure all for,
Want the best good effect,
Poor standard not acceptable,
Notable product rated category,
Number of stars more the better,
Definite decision decided,
Won't accept less up to standard,
Complete full load all aboard,
Want the best nothing less,
Judged as useful compliable,
Compatible use the lot,
Waste at a minimum,
High standard pure,
Good name retained,
Pertained paramount importance,
Regulation regulated,
Relgegation not accepted,
For the best forget the rest,
Inacceptable conquest,
Plausible definite doable,
Remain on right side for good.

COILED SPRING

Touchy or what!
My patience has run out,
Keep your distance "warning",
I'm wound up ready to explode,
All this potential wasted on trivia,
Waste of time can't combine refine,
All idiots make me seethe can't breathe,
Little devils belittle spittle noncommittal,
Could if I maybe should? Shouldn't I,
Death defies quantify gone awry wrong,
Wound up too tightly God almighty,
English blighters' contributors,
Causing problems bad relations,
Friendly selfish subscription,
Annual fee due don't really want to,
Committed can't get out of internment,
Regular regulation causes assimilation,
Pretentious importance implied implicates,
Preposterous imperative denied promptly.

GOT MY HEART

Something I really wanted to do,
But really wasn't qualified a hobby,
Build a sailing dinghy,
I had seen my dad build a kit,
Sailing boat assembling parts,
Even then as a boy was entranced,
If my dad could it, I could!
This gave me the general idea,
Of how to assemble and glue,
Kit of parts entranced me the smell of it,
Dad helped me make a start,
Once I had got underway,
There seemed a logical format,
Tentatively applied surely,
If it looked alright usually was,
Mistakes made changed,
I was loving it really somebody,
Professional profession personally,
I put my heart and soul into the job,
It proved plain sailing loving doing,
The smell of wood glue stuck on it,
The complete job made me proud,
Easy for the usurper.

TIME IS SLIPPING

Invisible unaccountable, gone,
Don't panic happens all the time,
Busy daily routine set clear,
Orderly order doing usual,
Kick starting in to play,
Off to a good start is an art,
List of ideas to be crossed off,
Once done moving forward,
Assembling building scene set,
Next job put in place arrange,
Set my own deadlines refined,
Getting on now knowing what to do,
A lot boring but must pursue,
Productive procedure produces,
Got others to help paid fair,
Employed correct skill trusted,
Being a boss assertive directive,
Saves me time held all mine,
Grasped gained pertained,
Promising promise promptly.

UP WITH NEW

There's pressure to keep coming up with new,
Whether that's self-inflicted or perceived,
Keeping in line with fellow friends aspiring,
Always to go one better competition for others,
Its not a race just haste without loss of face,
Competition to me is fun challenging reprimanding,
Setting the pace not worrying about trouble,
Adventuring into new ground often profound,
Raising the game setting sights higher,
Taking risks with a flyer multiplier,
Contriver complicates navigates around,
New ground is found by changing sounds,
Higher lowers expand grower bestower,
Give or take on the make borrow steal,
Thieve give to the poor, Robin hoods candour,
Intricate implicate intrinsic up against,
Which side of the fence makes sense,
With all diligence comprehend,
Spent up won't do nothing new,
Keeping up with the Jones's out of pocket.

GET IT RIGHT

Trying my best to be correct,
Standards are set morally obliged,
Have been taught to comply,
Should happen naturally,
Easy conformity applied,
Going along singsong,
Expecting comforting,
Same again retain,
Billed first hard fact,
Questionable amount,
More than expected,
Verble quotation doesn't figure,
Vague estimate exceeded,
Now must haggle,
Costs implausible,
Firm stance against,
Quoted estimate,
Vague excuse,
Get real,
Harboured spiel.

WHOLE GAMUT

Fully open everything exposed,
Symbolises the lot,
Leaving nothing out,
Holistic summary,
Fully inclusive retained,
Large family of similar,
Perpetuating purpose,
Inclusive inclusion,
Under no delusion,
Derivative derived,
Conceived contrived,
Waiting to yearn,
Apology affirmed,
Soulful soul,
Scored own goal,
End to end display,
Never say die,
Decent decency,
All things considered,
Controlling control,
Left out annulled,
Taken related,
All scenes navigated.

RAW EDGE

Sometimes it can prove real,
Element of newness,
Not overbaked cooked,
Something over rehearsed,
Pretentious not seen before,
Element of potential failure,
Could happen anytime,
New fashion style,
Put together in a hurry,
It won't last long,
Would stand improvement,
First take,
Loose edges,
Needs pulling together,
Harsh unforgiven,
Spent source,
Collective abandoned,
Real feel,
Brand new,
First play,
Not done before,
No history,
Acted out,
Rough job.

SAVING GRACE

Is my independence to think,
About anything listen,
To radio song expressing,
Rapping talking singing,
Point of view noise ring true,
Rhythms played again,
Similar verse repeating,
Dubbed over and over,
Slightly different innocence,
Coming around again,
Fully aware doing,
Change pursuing,
Solid flexible,
Correct inevitable,
Allows newness,
To old borrowed,
Unfolded unfurled,
Opening new world,
Of ideas to pursue,
Correct candour.
Couldn't ask for more,
Saving grace and face.

ART SPACE

Privileged position to use,
Respectfully used in turn,
Presence of mind shows,
Attitude view represented,
After collated one another,
Arrogant to give advice,
Personal freedom important,
Don't impose impositions,
Or regulate regulations,
Apprehend apprehensions,
Correspond correspondence,
Respectful reverence,
Due or undue,
Harness materials,
That aren't immaterial,
Friendly convivial,
Lively liveable,
Ideas conceivable,
Concerning concepts,
Accepting dialects,
Different differences,
Deviate deviations,
Artful diligence comprehends,
Precise compositions.

ALL IN THE PLANNING

Finding all the details is paramount,
To set plan in place,
Contingencies affect order,
Of play and delivery,
Just one thing makes changes,
Upsetting the balance,
Knock on effect affects,
Leaving one thing out,
Drawing in compensation,
Loss is assimilated,
Making up for change,
Weighing up rearrange,
Probable candidate stands out,
Could be better this competed,
For position of place,
It's a team effort finalising,
Contributions come into play,
Dismissing inefficient work,
That doesn't affect direct.
Solution is to be with it,
Play a part be a part of,
Sound planning sum of parts.

CONSIDERATION

Always a lot to take on board to get moving,
Matter of facts to set straight,
Once asserted leave dependants behind,
On their own to moan don't condone,
Regularity sets a parity once again,
Trying to get away from usual expected,
Labelled not a robot all that stuff,
Trying to make something new happen,
Making space for ideas to evolve,
Trying out testing fortuitus lucky,
Chances taken anticipation,
Hopeful for good return learnt,
Usually people respond in favour,
Fortunately, enough have got ways,
To confidently portray impartial advance,
Calculated risks taken a good chance,
I'll get reciprocation to back up what,
I've entered considerate consideration.

OTHERS' POINT OF VIEW

Music selected by others their favourite,
Was unusual in a roundabout way,
Their selection was down beat new,
Rhythm stuttered with a return,
Soulful lyrics moan condones,
Putting wrong to rights,
Opinion said fled tread,
Back again refrain,
Rolling along with aplomb,
Different rang true,
Drum and base fast deep,
Vocals on top peek trill,
Over and above what I'm used to,
Music has made me think widely,
Expanded my mind of a kind,
Taken to another place trace,
Tapping rapping convoluting,
Didn't see this coming strumming,
Foreign input funky strut,
Want to see others true.

OCCUPIED MIND

Always seem busy doing routine thinking,
Got to be healthy seeking out using,
Bit of initiative being creative,
Valuing the cost of shopping list,
What's important needed replace,
Do without upgrade shopping list,
Open minds change useful look,
Forward to providing new way,
Of making alternative directive,
That isn't vital but useful rearranged,
Order of doing place placement,
Got to think about this could work,
These needs changing out of use,
Get with it drop old fashioned,
Not just being trendy fashionable,
My mission is to see what's on the market,
Open to change my mind, assess better,
Busybody thinking organising order,
The power of mind over matter matters.

KEEP IN TOUCH WITH THE DIGITAL WORLD

Got to be a part of this modern language,
Details records all transcripted,
Acknowledged private passwords,
To make private personal singular,
To avoid theft from bank-robbers,
Corrupt corruption derelictions,
Avoid imposed affliction asserted,
My word you must watch your back,
You can't trust anybody so watch it,
Crafty devils deceive. Devious, Stealing,
Everything comes down to a dot- dot dash,
Binary numeric morse code tapped out,
Digital Pixel number one nought adds up,
To two and more all four repeating ten,
Multiples adding up squares calculating,
Equations calculus one plus one two,
Dodgy emails carried piggy back on another,
Access my computer intercepting fraud,
Too easy to be ignored digital deplored.

TOO MUCH

An expression of gratitude appreciation,
I used to use it too liberally trendy,
Thought I was being with it cool,
It made me assess normal dialect,
Over the top descriptive dictum,
Figure of speech trying to reach out,
Friendly commend recommend pretend,
Get with it over complicit join accepted,
Pretentious pressure over the top tip top,
Humour delicate balance might offend,
Carry it off out of fashion seen,
Want to be seen as part of party,
Friendly hearties declare share,
Convivial compliments complicate,
Only an expression all reckon with,
Plausible don't deny the comply.

REVISITED

Old haunt from ages ago held high,
From childhood memories stood,
Back intime memories rewind,
Physical structure still the same,
Water and sailing club showing age,
Water is water treated for drinking,
Boats floating surface tension held,
Archimedes' principal buoyancy upheld,
Floating on top in gravity allowing,
Correct principal applies floats,
Taking the weight ship-shape,
Recycled evaporated rain,
Clouds hold pertain purification,
Life's cycle reinvigorated again,
Simple true to life growth earths troth,
Giver receiver common dominator,
Appealing revealing user using,
Back and forth is its worthy solution,
Liquid solution to invigoration revisited.

ELEMENTAL

Affected by the weather,
Sun has gone in clouded over,
Moisture in the air heavy,
I can feel it in my bones,
Trudging feet tripping over,
Aching joints rheumatic pain,
Lost my bright and breezy,
Such a change under said,
Difference is dramatic,
Thespian apologetic,
Help seems distant,
Myself if I could,
Heavy eyes despised,
Under the weather,
Don't feel clever,
Turn for the worst,
Ready to burst,
Aching making, real not faking,
Disturbed hesitating,
Simple recreating,
Not relating complicating.

ABSTRACTION

Ephemeral not concrete hard to understand,
Wishy washy pretentious irregular no form,
No application or matter doesn't matter,
Hard to understand not normal defunct,
Has its own appeal intrinsic shocking shit,
Taken leave of all senses unregulated,
Not conforming to order nonsense,
Irregular proliferation pathetic limp,
Aesthetic intrinsic subjective happening,
Get real communication no appeal,
Relentless pretentious no structure,
Don't you get it? Its life no order,
No harm done diddle -dum conundrum,
Anything could happen let it unravel,
Continual drivel beautiful to some,
Reasonable reason of no reason,
Complete waste of time sublime,
Intrinsic personal subliminal,
Relying on unreliable trouble,
Conviction convoluted polluted,
Harassed confused nonsensical,
Many factions to legitimate jurisdiction,
Evolved in an unnatural order,
Only makes sense to friends,
Senseless condition affirmation,
A reason to ridiculous reason.

www.ingramcontent.com/pod-product-compliance
Lightning Source LLC
Chambersburg PA
CBHW071916070526
44583CB00016B/2019